# Contents

## Why this pack was developed

This pack has been developed for people who hear voices. It attempts to:

- give the facts about how many people hear voices, and what types of voices are most common
- offer a brief outline of theories about what causes voices, including a cognitive behavioural explanation
- reduce feelings of isolation and fear
- increase your understanding of your voice/s
- suggest cognitive behavioural methods for coping with hearing voices
- provide contact details for organisations and further reading, that may be helpful.

It may also be helpful for your family members, friends or carers to read the booklet.

Please feel free to photocopy the worksheets you'll find throughout this publication.

## Why should I try the pack?

This pack presents a cognitive behavioural approach and aims to help you develop new ways of coping with hearing voices. Some research has been undertaken which shows definite differences between people who cope with their voices and people who don't. People who are able to cope feel stronger and have more positive voices. Their voices are less authoritative and important. They are more able to set limits on their voices, and listen selectively to their voices. They talk more often about their voices, to people who they trust.

hearing voices

hearing voices

# Background

Many people feel they are alone in the experience of hearing voices. This can make you feel more anxious, fearful or upset. Consequently, you may try to ignore your voices, avoid situations where they occur, or not share your experiences with anyone else. Accepting and talking about your voices with people you trust can help you understand your experiences, reduce feelings of isolation, and increase your activity and enjoyment of life.

Hearing voices may actually be a more common experience than you think. Studies in America[1] suggest that 4-5 per cent of people hear voices at any one time. Many people hear voices at some point in their life, and do not necessarily receive a psychiatric diagnosis. Hearing voices may be understood in different ways depending on cultural background; for example, in Nigeria, hearing voices is thought to be possession by spirits. Throughout the ages, many famous people have claimed that they have heard voices. These include Socrates, Moses, Joan of Arc, Mohammed, Jesus, Carl Jung, Ghandi, Zoë Wannamaker (TV actress) and Anthony Hopkins (film actor). It is not necessarily hearing voices that is the problem, but rather the way we cope with them.

## What the voices say

Everyone's voices will be different, but there may be some similarities. Voices may appear to come from behind you, from the television or radio, from neighbours or people in the street, through the walls, or out of thin air. They may be loud or quiet; there may be many voices or only one. Some people recognise their voices, others do not. Some people understand their voices as being from God, Satan or a supernatural force.

Voices can say all sorts of things. They may be funny or abusive, comforting or frightening. Sometimes they talk about you or people around you. They may seem to say your thoughts out loud, or comment on what you are doing. They may talk about how you are feeling. They may seem to tell you what to do, say or think. Some people find it difficult to resist doing what their voices tell them, but it is important to remember that your voices cannot make you do anything. It is up to you if you respond to your voices or act on what they say.

Your voices may appear to be 'all knowing'. They may make it difficult to concentrate on conversations, work or activities. You may be unsure where they are coming from. Asking other people if they can hear the voices or trying to tape record them may be helpful. We will consider methods that you may find helpful when trying to cope with hearing voices, later in the booklet.

You may find it helpful to spend some time thinking about your voices in more detail. Recording details about your voices on paper or tape may be useful in learning more about your voices. The record sheet on the next page includes some questions that you may find of use to start thinking about your voices. Learning more about your voices, and why this can be helpful, will be considered in more detail later on.

**[1] Romme M. & Escher S.1996, 'Empowering People who hear voices', chapter 8 in Haddock G and Slade PD (eds) 1996, *Cognitive Behavioural Interventions with Psychotic Disorders*, London, Routledge; and Moore W. 2000, 'Talking Heads', *Observer magazine*, May 21 pp 45-6.**

## Thinking about my voices

| **Date/time** | **Description of voice/s**<br>e.g. gender, name, volume, age, quantity | **What the voice/s said**<br>Was it positive or negative? | **Situation**<br>Where, with whom? | **How I felt**<br>e.g. happy, anxious, scared. |
|---|---|---|---|---|
| | | | | |

## Common situations when people hear voices

People hear voices for lots of different reasons and in lots of different situations. Some of these may include:

- going off to sleep
- being stopped from sleeping
- using drugs like cocaine (coke, rocks, Charlie) or amphetamine (speed, whizz)
- in severe deprivation, for example, in a desert with no water
- when experiencing severe depression or psychosis; for example, schizophrenia
- with some physical illnesses, particularly if you have a high fever
- after very stressful events or prolonged trauma such as accidents, torture or violent attacks
- after being isolated for a long time, perhaps in the dark or away from others (some level of sensory deprivation); for example, in long-distance yachting or exploration, or in a hostage situation
- following bereavement, separation or divorce.

## Why and how do voices happen?

Finding an explanation, and so giving meaning to your experience of hearing voices, helps you to develop coping strategies. You may already have some thoughts on what you think causes your voices. There is no one single cause or explanation for why people hear voices.

There are many theories about why people hear voices. Some people think there is some kind of problem or abnormality in the development of the brain. They think this happens if a person experiences trauma whilst they are being born, or has a viral illness shortly after birth. Some people think voices occur due to problems in the development of personality. Perceiving things in an unusual way, such as problems in the way you think or understand experiences, or in the way messages are passed around your brain are also some reasons suggested for why people hear voices. There are some theories that people who hear voices have an abnormal blood flow to particular areas of their brain. Some doctors think that there is some kind of imbalance in chemicals in the brain, particularly that there may be too much of a chemical called dopamine. There is also thought to be a genetic component; that means that if you have a close family relative who hears voices, you are more likely to hear voices also.

It is common for people who hear voices to also have problems with their mood. You may have times when you feel very happy or very sad. Brain scans of people who hear voices have shown that when the voices are talking, there is activity in the area of the brain that is involved in speech – quite literally, voices are 'inner speech'. Some people believe voices start after emotional or psychological trauma, unresolved conflict, or understand them as having a religious, supernatural or mystical origin. The way you understand your voices will depend on what is normal experience for you.

Hearing voices can be influenced by a variety of factors. Stressful life events might act as a 'trigger' in people who are predisposed, or are likely, to hear voices. If you react to situations or problems by becoming stressed, you are more vulnerable. Other factors which may influence you hearing voices are a difficult family life, and having a chaotic lifestyle with no daily routine. Factors that may have a helpful effect on voices include having a daily routine, being active in coping with hearing voices, and developing your own understanding of your voices.

If you think hard about the situations you are most often in when you hear voices, you may be able to identify things that happen that are positive, even if hearing voices in itself is upsetting. For example, you may find that people pay more attention to you when you hear voices, and you may enjoy this.

You may want to spend some time thinking about where you think your voices come from. Do any of the factors talked about above relate to you or your experience? If the answer is 'yes', you may find it helpful to find out more information about them. Information is available from the organisations listed at the end of this handout, and there is a list of suggested further reading. If you are involved with any mental health workers, you may find it helpful to discuss this with them. You may have other ideas about where your voices come from. The table overleaf may help you to think about this. If you find writing difficult for any reason, you may want to make a recording, or ask a friend or carer to help.

## Where do my voices come from?

| **Date/time** | **Situation** Where, with whom? | **Voice/s heard** | **Where the voice/s came from** | **Evidence to support this** (use the information on pages 5-6 to help you) | **Life events which have been or are currently significant to your voice/s** |
|---|---|---|---|---|---|
| | | | | | |

# The cognitive behavioural approach

## What is cognitive behaviour therapy (CBT)?

Cognitive behaviour therapy, or CBT for short, is a way of understanding psychological problems. A commonly used model looks at three different areas. These are cognitions (thoughts), physical and emotional symptoms, and behaviour.

Our experiences in early life lead us to develop views of ourself, the world and other people. From this point, we develop personal rules about how to behave. A critical incident or trigger may cause us to have negative thoughts and start a cycle, linking those thoughts to emotions and physical symptoms, and causing us to behave in a particular way. CBT is based on the idea that a person's feelings and behaviour are a response to their beliefs. They are not fate, or unavoidable consequences.

## How does CBT explain my voices?

CBT works on the idea that there are links between life events and hearing voices. The types of life experiences a person has will effect what their voices say. The voices usually say things that are particularly relevant to the person who hears them. They often talk about a problem the person has that has not been solved; or about emotions relating to a past trauma; or secret fears. The cycle below shows how the experience of hearing voices is understood using CBT. It shows an example from a person who hears nasty voices, and how their voices and distress may be kept going. It includes life stresses in this to show how they can have an effect.

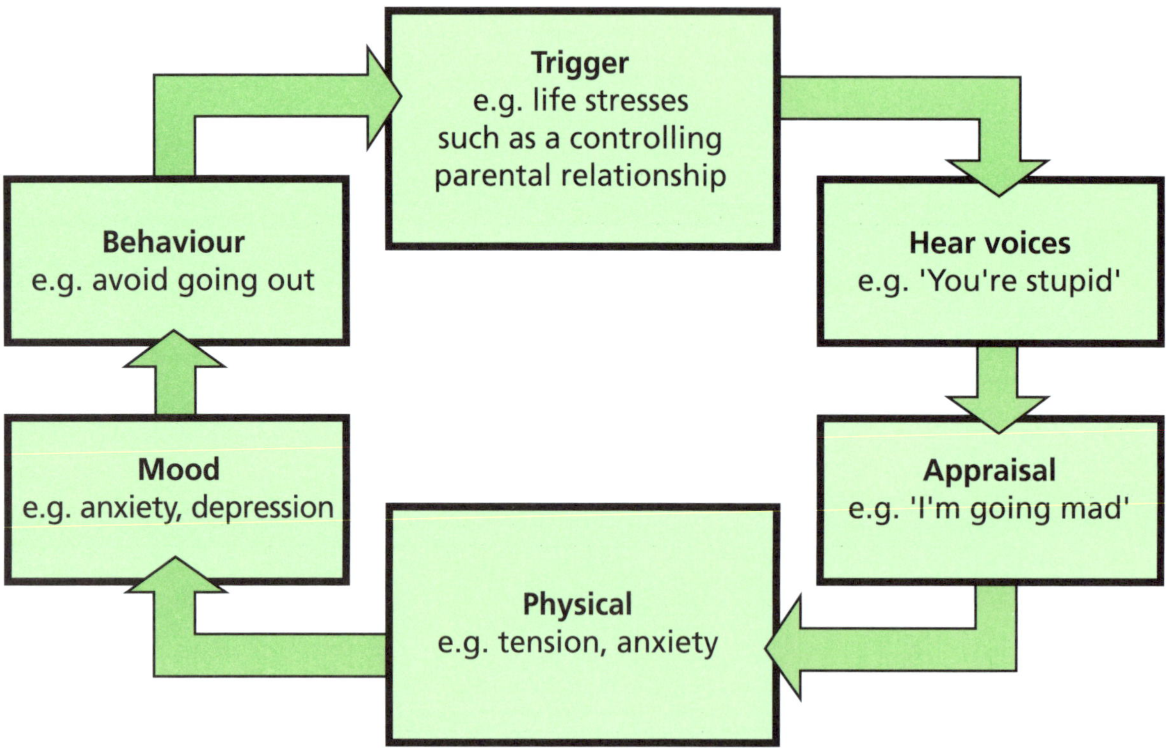

## The effects of stress

Another way to think about how stress and your personal likelihood of hearing voices is linked, is to think about you having a stress reservoir or lake. The banks of the lake are your stress threshold - the point at which you are unable to cope. There are various ways in which the stress levels of the lake can be filled.

We all have a level of day-to-day stress from home life, work, paying bills, family and so on. This stress can cause the level in the lake to go up and down.

The next layer may be related to ongoing problems that cause extra stress specific to you, like being ill or having an argument with a family member. This fills your lake up with water, but it doesn't quite overflow.

If a big event occurs, like moving house or being seriously ill, and your lake is already full, it seems like a rain cloud has come along and caused your lake to overflow.

This is when problems can happen. It may be when you first hear voices, and it is when your stress lake is full or overflowing in the future, that you are more likely to hear voices again. Learning to reduce your day-to-day stress and learning new ways of coping with your voices can help you reduce the water levels in your lake.

hearing voices

hearing voices

# How people behave when they hear voices

There are three main ways in which people will behave when they hear voices:

- **Engagement** describes behaviour such as listening to and responding to voices; doing things that bring on your voices.
- **Resistance** describes behaviours that help you avoid, or try to escape contact with your voices, such as distraction or shouting at the voices.
- **Indifference** is when you try not to engage with the voices: that is, to not respond at all.

CBT focuses on what the voices say and the relationships between you and your voices. It also looks at the types of problems you have in your daily life as a result of the voices, and how you might cope with them.

If your voices are mean or unpleasant, you are more likely to experience negative emotions (fear, depression, anxiety). If they are kind, you are more likely to feel positive emotions (humour, happiness, reassurance). You can use the Belief About Voices Questionnaire (BAVQ) to help you classify what type of voices you hear.

## Belief About Voices Questionnaire (BAVQ)

### How do you feel about your voice/s?

(Tick all that apply)

- [ ] My voice is punishing me for something I have done.
- [ ] My voice wants to help me.
- [ ] My voice is persecuting me for no good reason.
- [ ] My voice wants to protect me.
- [ ] My voice is evil.
- [ ] My voice is helping to keep me sane.
- [ ] My voice wants to harm me.
- [ ] My voice is helping me to develop my special powers or abilities.
- [ ] My voice wants me to do bad things.
- [ ] My voice is helping me to achieve my goal in life.
- [ ] My voice is trying to corrupt or destroy me.
- [ ] I am grateful for my voice.
- [ ] My voice is very powerful.
- [ ] My voice reassures me.
- [ ] My voice frightens me.
- [ ] My voice makes me happy.
- [ ] My voice makes me feel down.
- [ ] My voice makes me feel angry.
- [ ] My voice makes me feel calm.
- [ ] My voice makes me feel anxious.
- [ ] My voice makes me feel confident.

### What do you usually do when you hear your voice?

- [ ] I tell it to leave me alone.
- [ ] I try and take my mind off it.
- [ ] I try and stop it.
- [ ] I do things to prevent it talking.
- [ ] I am reluctant to obey it.
- [ ] I listen to it because I want to.
- [ ] I willingly follow what my voice tells me to do.
- [ ] I have done things to start to get in contact with my voice.
- [ ] I seek the advice of my voice.

## How do you cope with your voices?

One of the first steps in coping with your voices is to learn more about them. We have already thought about the nature of voices, what they sound like and what they say. We have also spent some time thinking about where they come from. Think about the techniques that you use currently to cope when you hear voices. Are some methods more helpful or successful than others? Try making a list of your coping techniques below.

..........................................................................................................................................

..........................................................................................................................................

..........................................................................................................................................

..........................................................................................................................................

..........................................................................................................................................

..........................................................................................................................................

..........................................................................................................................................

..........................................................................................................................................

..........................................................................................................................................

..........................................................................................................................................

..........................................................................................................................................

..........................................................................................................................................

..........................................................................................................................................

..........................................................................................................................................

..........................................................................................................................................

..........................................................................................................................................

..........................................................................................................................................

..........................................................................................................................................

..........................................................................................................................................

..........................................................................................................................................

..........................................................................................................................................

..........................................................................................................................................

Now use the table overleaf to see how, and if, these techniques are working for you.

This booklet looks at methods of coping with hearing voices that are based on the CBT model. You may find by this stage that you are already using some of the coping techniques mentioned in this section. Hopefully there will be some that you haven't already tried! Remember, there is always more than one option for coping with any problem, and in the section 'Choosing the best way to cope' there is a diagram to help you consider your options and choose the one that suits you best.

## Coping with my voices

| Date/time | Situation | Voice/s heard | How I felt | Coping methods tried | How I felt after using coping method | How voices changed after using coping method |
|---|---|---|---|---|---|---|
| | | | | | | |

# Some coping techniques

## Learning more about your voices

Learning even more detail about your voices may help you understand them better, why they say what they do, and what factors effect them. You have already begun to learn more about your voices in earlier parts of the booklet. Using the spaces below, a separate piece of paper, or a recording, think about the following questions, and write down your response.

- What does the voice sound like?
- Do I recognise the voice/s?
- How many voices do I hear?
- How often do I hear them?
- Is the voice/s male or female?
- How old is the voice/s?
- What does the voice/s say?
- When did it start?
- What is my understanding of where the voice comes from?
- Has the voice told you its identity? If not, how do you know who it is? Often people report hearing the voice of God or Satan. How do you know? Would God say the types of things your voice says?
- Do you believe the voice?
- Is the voice positive or negative?
- Do the voices comment, command or criticise?
- What makes the voice better or worse?
- How does hearing voices effect you? What does it help you do, or prevent you from doing? Do you get upset as a result of hearing voices?

The way you understand the identity and purpose of your voices is important because it has a big impact on the way you respond to your voices, how you behave, and how you feel.

## Recording the pattern of your voices

Keeping a record of your voices, when and where they occur may help you identify patterns. This may help you be better prepared for when they occur, and to use different ways of coping in different situations. The diary sheet on the following page may help you in this process. You may also find it helpful to ask a family member or friend to help you with this. Try completing the sheet for the next two weeks, at least, to find out more about the patterns of your voices.

If you feel your voice comes from somewhere outside yourself, involving a friend or relative who you trust at this stage may be helpful. If your voice/s do come from an external source then your friend or relative should also be able to hear it. If they can't, you may want to consider why this is the case.

## The pattern of my voices

| **Date/time** | **Voice/s heard** | **What the voice/s said** | **My mood was...** | **Situation**<br>Where, who with, doing what? | **My reaction or coping method** |
|---|---|---|---|---|---|
| | | | | | |

## Testing your beliefs

**James felt that his voices were coming from somewhere outside of himself and that if others said they couldn't hear, it was because they were lying. He agreed to try to tape record the voice next time he heard it and when he listened to the tape he agreed he could not hear the voice. James then suggested that perhaps the messages brought by the voice were intended just for him and that this was why others could not hear the voice. He used a piece of paper with two columns – 'For' and 'Against' – to explore the evidence for this. He then looked at how his voices changed – what situations made them worse or better. In this way, James came to the conclusion that his voices were a part of himself coming from inside his mind.**

Using cognitive behavioural methods, you can test your beliefs about your voices in a systematic, step-by-step way. This may help you adapt or dispute your beliefs, and so relieve any distress you feel as a result of hearing voices. The techniques may also help you to change your behaviour or response to your voices, and ultimately reduce your overall experience of hearing voices. Think about what your voices say. If they make statements rather than giving you a general 'running commentary', think about how much you believe what they say. Try rating your belief out of 100 per cent. You may find it helpful to use the form on the next page to think about other explanations or responses to your voices.

You may find it helpful to write down statements that you use to challenge what your voices say. An example has been included on the sheet overleaf to help you.

You may find it helpful to tape record your responses to your voices when they are not active, then replay the tape when your voices are active. Write down what happens. For example, if your voices often tell you that you are a bad person, try recording responses like, "I am a good person. My friends [use their names] tell me that they like me, and they would not choose to spend time with me if they didn't like me. I don't break the law, or do anything that hurts or upsets anyone else". Listen to these responses when your voices are active, and see what happens.

If your voices tell you what to do, you may want to try behaving against them. Write down what you think will happen, and then what actually does happen. For example, if your voices tell you to throw something like furniture or ornaments, write down what you think will happen if you don't do it. Then try to resist throwing the object, and write down what actually does happen. Were you right in your prediction? How do you feel having resisted doing what your voices were telling you to do? Could you try this in another situation?

## Testing my beliefs

| Date/time | Voice/s heard | What they said | Percentage belief (0-100 per cent) | Evidence for/against alternative view | Percentage belief evidence (0-100 per cent) | **Outcome** e.g. changes to mood or behaviour/ coping skills |
|---|---|---|---|---|---|---|
| 6/12/02 8am | One male, called Red | I am a bad person and deserve to be alone. Nobody likes me. I am stupid and people talk about me when I am not there. | 85 per cent | I haven't done anything wrong or committed any crime. I saw a friend yesterday and people at college talk to me. The teacher says I am doing well so I can't be that stupid. | 30 per cent | Feel a bit better, less worried and a bit happier. I think I will talk to my nurse about this, next visit. I will plan to do something nice today. |

## Attentional control

This refers to the process of taking control over how much attention you pay to your voices, and when. This is quite a difficult skill, and may take some time to master. You may try ignoring the voice/s or giving them attention at specific times. You may even contract with your voice/s that you will communicate with them for a set period of time at a pre-arranged time of day. Alternatively, you may find it helpful to ignore your voice/s. For example, there may be a particular time of day when it is more convenient to listen to your voices, say between five and six o'clock in the evening. You may tell your voices that you will give them your attention between these times, but that if they speak to you at any other time, you will ignore them. This process may take some practice, and you may try a few different ways of doing this before you find one that works best for you, and fits in with your lifestyle.

### Problem solving

Some people find it helpful to focus on a particular problem or goal they have that is not necessarily related to hearing voices and set about trying to resolve it. For example, if you want to learn a new skill, how you might go about achieving it. There is a more detailed explanation of problem solving at the end of the handout in the section 'Choosing the best option', with an example based on how to choose the most helpful way for you to cope with your voices.

## Distraction

Using ways of distracting yourself, such as listening to music or the radio, or watching television, may help reduce your voice/s. Some people find this method is more effective if they use headphones. Other activities such as playing a musical instrument, writing your experiences down, painting or reading, may also help.

## Physical activity

Changing your level of activity may help. If you have followed earlier stages of the handout, you may have discovered patterns to your experience of hearing voices. If they are worse when you are inactive, increasing physical activity, like going for a walk or gardening, may help. Physical activity is also known to increase the level of 'feel-good' chemicals in your body. Opposite to this, some people find their voice/s get worse when they try to do too much, or are over-stimulated. Taking some time out, resting and spending some time in a quiet, calm environment or having a warm bath may help at these times.

## Indulgence

Treating yourself to something you enjoy may help you cope with the voices, or help you to associate them with positive experiences. Eating or drinking favourite foods and drinks are an example of this. You may want to use indulgence as a means of rewarding yourself when you have coped well with distressing voices. Some people may include smoking in this category, although it is important to note the physical health risks posed by smoking. Treats are very individual, it is important that you indulge yourself, but not so excessively so that it causes other problems.

## Socialisation

This refers to how much contact you have with other people, and depends on what patterns your voice/s follow. You may find it helpful to increase your contact with other people when you have difficulty coping with your voice/s, and may seek out company. Others may want to withdraw when voice/s are particularly difficult, and spend some time on their own.

## Talking

Talking to a friend or relative may be helpful at times when you are finding it difficult to cope with your voices. Others may find it helpful to talk to somebody of a more anonymous nature, for example, with a mental health helpline or Samaritans.

## Activity scheduling

This is related to physical activity. Some people find that hearing voices leaves them feeling tired and with little energy or motivation. This is another area where CBT may be helpful. Activity scheduling is a way of coping by carefully structuring what kinds of things you are going to do each day. It is important to be realistic and to start with small, achievable steps. Try rating each activity you do, based on: mastery (how far you achieve the activity) and pleasure (how much you enjoy the activity). The table on the next two pages may be used to help you, and includes an example given by a person who had been working with this technique with the author.

## Activity schedule

M = Mastery, P = Pleasure. Score both on scale: 0.....1.....2.....3.....4.....5.....6.....7.....8
O = No achievement at all/no enjoyment, 8 = completely achieved, extremely enjoyable.

| | Monday (example) | Monday | Tuesday | Wednesday | Thursday | Friday | Saturday | Sunday |
|---|---|---|---|---|---|---|---|---|
| **7-8am** | asleep | | | | | | | |
| **8-9am** | asleep | | | | | | | |
| **9-10am** | asleep | | | | | | | |
| **10-11am** | Got up, had breakfast M=5, P=2 | | | | | | | |
| **11-12am** | Had shower M=4, P=3 | | | | | | | |
| **12-1pm** | Watched TV M=8, P=6 | | | | | | | |
| **1-2pm** | Nurse visited M=8, P=5 | | | | | | | |
| **2-3pm** | Went to shop M=6, P=2 | | | | | | | |
| **3-4pm** | Walked dog M=8, P=6 | | | | | | | |
| **4-5pm** | Watched TV M=7, P=5 | | | | | | | |
| **5-6pm** | Had dinner M=7, P=3 | | | | | | | |
| **6-7pm** | Went to college class M=6, P=7 | | | | | | | |

| | Monday (example) | Monday | Tuesday | Wednesday | Thursday | Friday | Saturday | Sunday |
|---|---|---|---|---|---|---|---|---|
| **7-8pm** | College class M=6, P=7 | | | | | | | |
| **8-9pm** | Visited friend M=8, P=6 | | | | | | | |
| **9-10pm** | Went home M=7, P=2 | | | | | | | |
| **10-11pm** | At home alone M=8, P=1 | | | | | | | |
| **11-12pm** | Watched TV M=6, P=1 | | | | | | | |
| **12-1am** | Watched TV M=6, P=1 | | | | | | | |
| **1-2am** | Watched TV M=5, P=1 | | | | | | | |
| **2-3am** | Went to bed M=7, P=2 | | | | | | | |
| **3-4am** | Asleep | | | | | | | |
| **4-5am** | Asleep | | | | | | | |
| **5-6am** | Asleep | | | | | | | |
| **6-7am** | Asleep | | | | | | | |

## Anxiety management

Some people find the experience of hearing voices frightening, particularly at first. Anxiety or stress that occurs naturally as we go through life can also make voices worse. Anxiety may result in voice/s being louder, more frequent or more negative in nature. Hyperventilation, a fairly common symptom of anxiety, has been suggested as precipitating, or setting off, voices. As a result, some people find it helpful to learn more about anxiety and how to manage it. You may want to consider anxiety management courses or reading material. Further information about courses offering this may be obtained from your GP, mental health worker, local library or college. The organisations listed at the end of the booklet may also be able to offer further advice.

## Relaxation

Relaxation tapes or exercises may be helpful. People often feel anxious when they hear voices. As we talked about in the section 'How does CBT explain my voices?', being generally less anxious in your day-to-day life can help you cope better with rises in anxiety when you hear voices, or in response to any life stress. Practising relaxation techniques on a daily basis can help you achieve an overall lower level of anxiety.

Using breathing techniques such as abdominal breathing may help you to feel calmer when you are in a stressful situation and so reduce the likelihood of hearing voices, or help you cope better if you do hear your voices.

Aromatherapy oils contained in bath products, scented candles, or for use in oil burners, are often used for relaxing and, again, may de-stress you to be better able to cope with your voices.

Further information may be obtained from your GP, mental health worker, or the organisations at the end of this handout. There are also some useful Mind booklets that may help you cope with feelings of anxiety and stress – see 'Further reading'.

# Choosing the best way to cope

Solving problems is part of our every day lives, but sometimes we can find it difficult, and spend time worrying rather than solving a problem with positive action. Choosing the best way to try to cope with hearing voices may seem difficult when you have lots of options to try. It is simply another problem to solve. The following four steps aim to help you choose the best option for you.

1. **State your problem**
   In this case, problems coping with hearing voices.

2. **State your target**
   Learning new ways to cope with hearing voices. Make sure your aim is realistic: you may be able to cope better with your voices; you may not be able to get rid of them altogether.

3. **List your options**
   Brainstorming can be helpful for doing this. Write down all the ideas that come into your head, no matter how daft they might seem. A few examples are shown below.

## Alternatives to coping with hearing voices

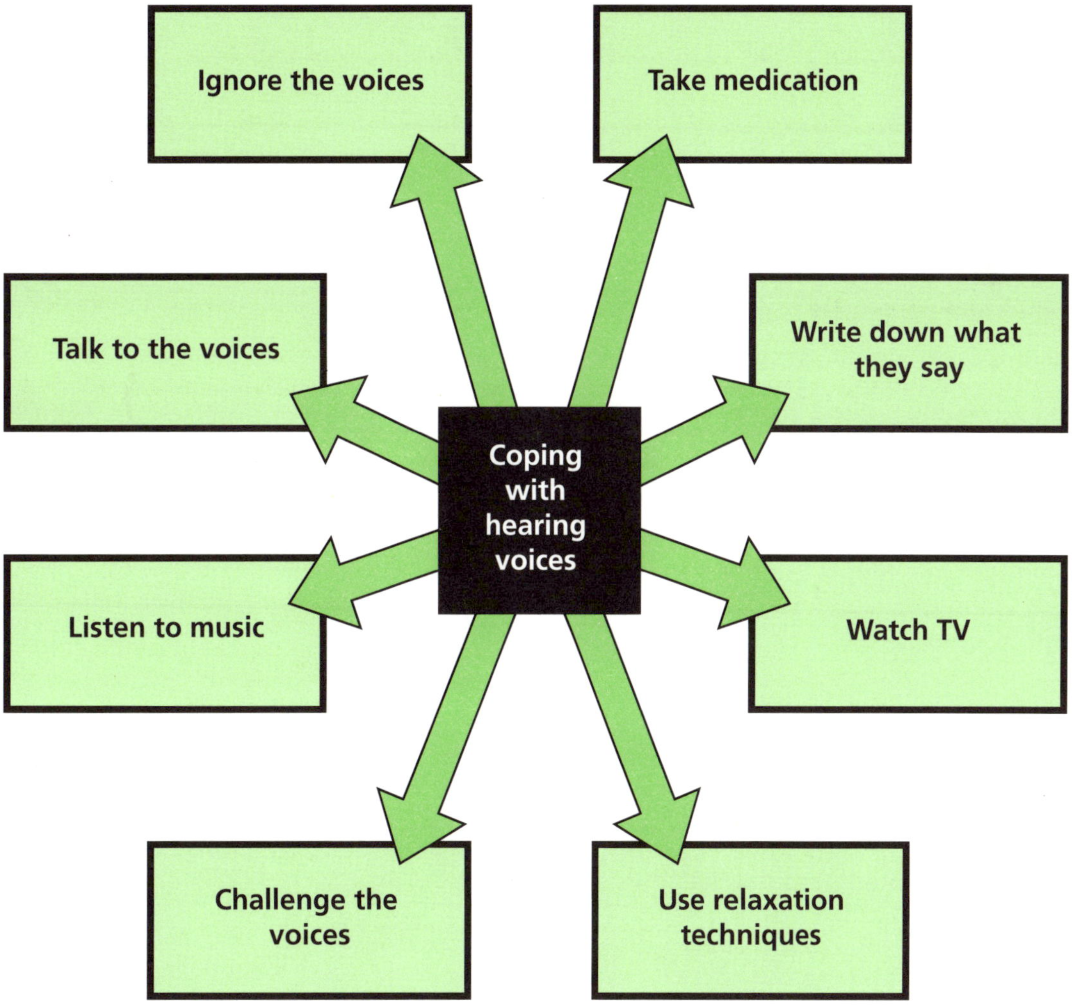

**4. Choose the best option for you**

The table below may help you decide. Try scoring each of your options, and then you can use the one that scores highest. If that doesn't work out, try the one with the next highest score.

| **Option: challenge the voices** (Example) | **Good** 3 points | **Alright** 2 points | **Bad** 1 point | **Total** |
|---|---|---|---|---|
| How does this make me feel? | | X | | |
| How does this effect others? | X | | | |
| Short-term gains | | X | | |
| Long-term gains | X | | | |
| Viability | | X | | |
| Sub totals | 6 | 6 | 0 | 12 |
| **Option:** | | | | |
| How does this make me feel? | | | | |
| How does this effect others? | | | | |
| Short-term gains | | | | |
| Long-term gains | | | | |
| Viability | | | | |
| Sub totals | | | | |
| **Option:** | | | | |
| How does this make me feel? | | | | |
| How does this effect others? | | | | |
| Short-term gains | | | | |
| Long-term gains | | | | |
| Viability | | | | |
| Sub totals | | | | |

Just beware, there are three kinds of problems:

- Those you can solve right now.
- Those you will be able to solve in time.
- Those which can't be solved.

Trying to solve problems that can't be solved is unhelpful, and can cause you a lot of unhappiness. If a problem is unsolvable, try to think about it as a fact. If it is a fact, then is it really a problem?